Preoperative Assessment in Hospitals and Clinics Low Complexity

Dr. Fernando Martín Correa

DEDICATION

"My gratitude to all my theachers who though me by example to work as anesthesiologist and specially my family who are the reason for my life".

CONTENT

THANKS

My thanks to my parents who are role models and values instilled in me; my
brothers and I love them as they are, truly, with golden heart and soul
transparent; my in-laws who are also family that is always unconditionally
through thick and thin; grandmother to Sofia still strong as an ox and finally
with all my heart, my lovely wife and son, who are the light that illuminates
your smile all the immensity, that make me happy, and thanks to them I am
the happiest man on earth.

Fernando Martín Correa

1 INTRODUCTION

The pre-operative assessment is an important part of our activities as doctors.

Anesthesiologists have taken the lead in defining the optimal and most cost effective method compared to the preoperative assessment, including the creation of systems that allow patients submitted to surgery in inpatient and outpatient settings in the best condition and with sufficient information available to provide the highest quality care.

The first concern is the safety of the patient and check that the complexity of the activity does not affect the care of the same.

The second is the physical and operational integrity of the system. In these events take place.

The American Society of Anesthesiologists (ASA) has a long and respected career for his work in establishing standards, guidelines, benchmarks and recommendations for exercise.

There is no formal definition of ASA in different types of practice: as an employee in a hospital of high complexity and low complexity.

The preoperative assessment is the essential element and start anesthesiologist outpatient procedure.

The type of practice, in hospital or added complexity should not affect the quality of the pre-anesthetic, agreed that valuation area is found, the contractor shall make use of their abilities to evaluate the patient and the surgical procedure to be performed without reducing the quality of care in a given patient.

Professional practice in hospitals and clinics low complexity should be more sensitive to issues related to personnel (decreased from the high complexity) and patient satisfaction.

The aim of this book is to determine the importance of pre-operative assessment in hospitals and medical clinics of low complexity, with the concern to provide anesthesia to the patient and check that the complexity of the activity does not affect the care of the same security.

2 TYPES OF PRACTICE

SENIOR FINANCIAL HOSPITAL COMPLEX

In general anesthesiologists are related to the main hospital facilities and multifaceted care centers where professionals from different specialties are present with immediate availability of diagnostic, therapeutic, and interclinical patient recovery assistance.

Probably the most serious patients requiring more support available.

The staff is made up of residents, technicians and graduates in anesthesia and medical anesthesiologists (at 2 or more) and 24-hour guard.

Part of the role of the physician is to teach residents to investigate new anesthetic techniques applied inside and outside the hospital.

The working relationship with the institution can vary from a contract with the university, hospital or clinic, so the doctor is the situation obtaining compensation through a monthly salary.

The desire to establish changes in the hospital will vary according to the political and economic competition with other services or departments for funds, materials, monitors, etc. force.

RETAIL FINANCIAL HOSPITAL COMPLEX

Doctors anesthesiologists can work in any type of institution but usually does in ambulatory surgical centers or smaller and smaller sub-specialization in hospitals that exercise more complex.

Auxiliary diagnostic methods are more basic: radiology, electrocardiography and blood and urine very general, and have minimal support in terms interconsultations with various professionals, diagnostic and therapeutic care and recovery.

Surgical and anesthetic procedures are generally more limited and less risky for patients.

The severity of the patient may be less by choice, including only the ASA 1 and 21 patients and referral of patients to a hospital complex or more complex clinical cases.

Staff can be only a physician, or a licensed physician and anesthesia technician and rarely, a doctor and two licensed or anesthesia technicians more space to the lack of staff for unhealthiness of it.

There is less budget for the anesthesia service because the hospital gives priority to other major clinical and basic as health, pediatrics, public health, etc. services.

Table 1 - Classification of the American Society of Anesthesiology patient surgical [1].

ASA Grade	Status	Absolute Mortality (%)
1	Normal healthy patient	0.1
2	Mild systemic disease, or patient over 80 years old	0.2
3	Systemic disease that causes definite functional limitation on life	1.8
4	Severe systemic disease that is a constant threat to life	7.8
5	Moribund patient unlikely to survive 24 hours without surgery	9.4

3 COMPONENTS FOR RECOMMENDATION ANESTHESIOLOGIST EXERCISE

PATIENT FACTORS

Several areas were identified.

The main point is the patients themselves and their general medical health. This review draws on conventional elements as directed history and physical examination, testing and consultation indicated relevant, and plan formulation anesthesia if the operation at that hospital is decided.

ADMINISTRACIÓN DE RECURSOS

One area was specifically identified the optimal resource management , which is in the general category of opportunity to pre- operative tests.

This section considers that other factors , such as socio- economic demographic, clinical condition of the patient and even location and nature and current status of the health service that govern the time the pre - anesthetic assessment should be performed .

Was also identified the type and degree of invasiveness of the procedure and medical risk to the patient impacted by the valuation process .

DEGREE OF INVASION OF SURGERY AND SEVERITY OF DISEASE

Two groups are easily distinguishable from surgical invasiveness : high and low.

And severity of the disease: high and low ; to generate a review .

Falls mature patients with high surgical invasiveness process and a very serious illness must be addressed at some point before surgery .

At the other end of the spectrum are patients with a low degree of surgical invasiveness and low severity of illness that require only be seen surgery.2 day .

The consequence of this is that the intensity of care should fit the physiological challenge of early surgery (neurological surgery compared with a sebaceous cyst in the arm) or the underlying physiology of the patient (for example, unstable angina compared with low pressure treated) . Must have the ability to discern and classify patients as long as providing the best care possible .

4 IMPACT OF SIZE

INSTALLATIONS OF HIGH COMPLEXITY

A big center likely justify formal clinical pre-anesthetic assessment.

There is a large caseload often complex.

The combination of many patients, the high degree of surgical invasion and severity of each patient each represent a factor that generates confusion.

There is a geometric increase in the risk of delay.

Delays can be overcome by changing other cases to the time available but yet this alters the system and the individual.

Center is likely to have many staff working at multiple sites, which increases the possibility that staff members are available on a regular basis to be part of a clinical pre-anesthetic assessment.

A large facility has greater range of operating room personnel at all times and thus is easier to accommodate delays.

INSTALLATIONS OF LOW COMPLEXITY

A small facility is more vulnerable to delays and postponements that great because there are fewer options to fill the time not used.

There may be fewer people available, including "after hours".

Vacation or illness may adversely impact the availability of coverage.

However, it is reasonable to assume that in a small facility is less likely that more complex procedures are performed at high-risk patients and therefore the number of possible delays will be reduced.

In small institutions is more likely that the delay is related to personnel problems because they often expect staff to work extra time to cover delays.

Fernando Martín Correa

5 ASSESSMENT REQUIREMENTS PRE-ANESTHESIA

ASA standards and guidelines [3-4] require the patient to undergo pre-anesthetic assessment.

They do not define the time such assessment should be performed, but identify the anesthesiologist is responsible for this part of the peri-anesthetic care.

Perhaps the right time for the pre-anesthetic assessment is the most critical element for effective care management.

A measure to all situations and should not adjust to.

An important part of the Practice Advisory for Preanesthesia Care refers to the right time, as mentioned above.

EVALUATION FACTORS OF PRE-ANESTHESIA

The pre-anesthetic assessment is an exercise in patient communication and coordination administered in the most effective way regarding cost possible resources.

It is a small community practice, especially where anesthesia care is given only by physicians, to find an opportune time to assess the patient can be difficult.

Patients do not like to wait until the end of the day, especially if they had a morning appointment with the surgeon.

Resources "after hours" as the diagnostic lab, might not be available except if required urgently. When other information is needed, the office or hospital department physician may be closed , requiring postpone the procedure , obtain the nearest surgery information and hope that no major problems or repeat a test that could have been done just a couple of weeks earlier.

The alternative that anesthesiologists assess patients during their normal working hours may not be practical .

The doctor cannot assess patients awaiting surgery unless you work as a team .

Seeing patients on a regular and predictable between cases will lead to rush the process and delay the operating room , causing everyone to be angry with the anesthesiologist.

In professional practice in hospitals with low complexity group exerted anesthesia usually is small or sole , the cancellation or delay of cases is directly related not only to income but to the quality of life if the delayed cases are conducted on a subsequent later service providers , surgeons, operating room staff , cleaners and sterilization , among others, that are necessary for the peri- operative care .

In addition , the family may be upset , especially if the cause of the delay was avoidable .

These conditions encourage the formation of an effective process for pre-anesthetic evaluation of patients .

THE ROAD

The pre-anesthetic assessment requires the interaction of several different groups: surgeons, anesthesiologists, clinical, other physicians, nurses, laboratory and diagnostic services, and administration.

All these actions take place around a person, the patient.

These activities can occur serially, although not necessarily always respecting the same sequence.

Roads and interaction sequence should be optimized and will vary according to each specific environment, but must be addressed.

PATIENT PROBLEMS

What is often not considered is the impact of these multiple visits or interviews with the patient and their support mechanisms.

For example , if a patient should go to the Regional Hospital of Caacupé (low complexity) for surgery, and lives in Streams and Estuaries , will take the best 4-6 hours to reach the hospital.

In the case of a 15-minute interview to the middle of the day , you will lose all day, even two days if attention is restricted by order of arrival costs related books when outside the home, and represent a significant burden .

Other concerns such as taking time off work , loss of income in the case of those who are self-employed , have a child or adult care , arranging transportation, lodging and meals or other items should be considered in determining overall "cost " of the pre - anesthetic assessment .

Resource conservation is beyond the hospital environment or operating room immediately , and should include costs for the patient.

STAFF

This is the key element.
Even the smallest surgical environment will benefit from having a subject whose task is to coordinate the pre -operative process, especially if a person committed .
The time you spend at your job will vary depending on the workload and the number of employees.
A small institution only require an individual every 24 hours.
The coordinate appointments (lab , interviews) so that patients must make multiple visits can not only improve the process.
It is unlikely that in this context of practice procedures are carried out in high-risk or high-risk patients .
So the anesthesiologist can see more patients more safely the day of surgery with a low probability of cancellation or delays for medical reasons.
A mechanism is needed to allow assessment by the anesthesiologist in questionable cases or if the patient wishes to speak with an anesthesiologist especially in particular.
In hospitals with low complexity perhaps the individual who coordinates the pre -anesthetic interview with responsibilities with other providers.
For example , you may need to be checked against the history and physical examination , record office, X ray studies colpocytology and cervix, etc.

* Anecdote: One day, I was a patient in the operating room for removal of a fatty tumor with local anesthesia. The fatty tumor was large and the surgeon does call for anesthesia guard and says, "Johnny, make a Ketalarcito (some ketamine for the patient to stay still), the technician does as requested by the surgeon and this continues to operate ... within 10 minutes the patient is re-moved and the surgeon repeats: "Juanito, make a Ketalarcito, the technician makes it Ketalarcito and the surgeon is still

operating ... spend a few minutes and the patient turns around and says: "Johnny, please do me a Ketalarcito".

6 METHODOLOGIES FOR THE DETECTION

An important element of the pre-operative assessment is a "review of systems" type questionnaire.

In face-to-face interview, most physicians have addressed several questions used to determine if the patient has other diseases, not necessarily related to the surgical procedure, which may impact anesthetic care.

This is formalized through a written questionnaire, which can be filled by the patient or by the interviewer and to suit the patient's language.

The questionnaires sent to patients before the interview, for example in the waiting room, can help gather information such as what medications you take and what the patient has suffered allergies and previous procedures, family history of malignant hyperthermia, especially if it is an old or requires the assistance of another person.

Assessment Questionnaire preoperative[5].

AGE:	WEIGHT:	HEIGHT:	GENDER:

ALLERGIES:	MEDICATION RECEIVING	SURGERIES THAT HAVE PERFORMED
1-	1-	1-
2-	2-	2-
3-	3-	3-
4-	4-	4-

	YES	NO	COMMENTS
YOU HAD ANESTHESIA EVER?			
YOU GOT A PROBLEM WITH IT?			
THE FAMILY HAD ANY?			
SMOKING? MANY PER DAY? HOW DO?			
HAVE COUGH?			
CAST OUT WHEN SOMETHING COUGHS?			
HAD OR HAVE ASTHMA?			
HE HAD PROBLEMS BREATHING?			
CLIMBING STAIRS WITHOUT YOU MISSED THE AIR?			
YOU HAVE MISSED THE AIR WHILE LYING?			
HAVE YOU EVER HAD ANY CHEST PAIN?			
HAD KIDNEY DISEASE?			
EVER PUT YELLOW?			
HAD HEPATITIS?			
HAD HIATAL HERNIA OR SUFFER HEARTBURN?			
CONSUME ALCOHOLIC BEVERAGES? HOW MUCH?			
HAD SEIZURES? HAD FAINTING?			
SUFFERING FROM HEADACHES OFTEN?			
HAD OR HAVE ARTHRITIS?			
FREQUENTLY SUFFER FROM BACK PAIN?			
OR HAVE HAD PROBLEMS THYROID?			
SUFFER ANY TREND HEMORRHAGIC?			
EVER HAD ANEMIA?			
CONSUME ASPIRIN? UNTIL WHEN?			
HAVE A LOOSE OR BROKEN TOOTH?			
HAVE A DENTAL PROSTHESIS?			
PROTESIS HAVE ANY?			
HAD PSYCHIATRIC ASSISTANCE?			

Only for women:

LAST MENSTRUAL DATE	CONTRACEPTIVE METHOD

Nº OF PREGNANCY	Nº OF ABORTIONS	LIVE CHILDREN	CHILDREN BORN DEAD

Other comments:

Informed Consent:

I received Dr. _____ the information on the procedures that I have to practice and the risks it entails.

All my questions were answered and authorize the performance of such procedures on me.

Name:
Identity Card No:
Address:
Phone:
Signature:

LEADERSHIP

Whatever the method selected for the pre-anesthetic assessment, which vary according to the specific needs and resources of each site, it is necessary that the anesthesiologist is involved in the process.

It is also important to remember that this is a medical assessment and not just a "list type" process.

Lists are efficient and effective to verify that a specific area or system are not overlooked, but the integration of information in the anesthetic plan is part of the medical duties of anesthesiologists with patient.

7 INTERROGATION AND PHYSICAL EXAMINATION

INTERROGATION

Although the patient count with a history, it is important to obtain information about a family history of importance (one of the most important is malignant hyperthermia) should be considered the habits of the patient to investigate any drug, type of anesthesia received to assess a difficult airway, and the reaction to certain drugs, it is necessary to investigate the nature of religion and the obstetric patient is predisposed to major bleeding and Jehovah's Witnesses refuse transfusions.[6]
The history of blood transfusion reactions and if any, as well as concomitant diseases, heart disease, hypertension, thyroid disease, etc.[7]

EXAMINATION PHYSICAL

It starts with determining the pathobiology general inspection of the patient, as well as alterations, including overweight (which can reach morbid obesity) or otherwise malnutrition in any degree, or edema is; facies, characteristics of the skin, conjunctiva and mucous membranes are determined, eg dermatitis, jaundiced, hydration, capillary refill and pallor, neck mobility and the characteristics of the trachea must be verified, and a thorough examination of the oral cavity comprising the maximum aperture of the mouth, presence of oropharyngeal and tonsillar infections, dental status.
When dentures are observed, should be complete, should be left in place because they maintain the normal anatomical configuration of the mouth, allowing a proper fit of the mask; in the case of partial dentures must be removed to avoid accidents.
For the anesthesiologist is particularly interesting to assess the airway in

17

pregnancy, because, in this situation difficult intubation has a low incidence, but significant, an assessment of the patient still needed with the simple and non-invasive methods to help us anticipate problems that may arise. Among them are:

1-   Classification of Mallampati modified by Samsoon and Young.[8,9]

      Which relates tongue size to the size of the oral cavity, it determines the extent to which the language allows to visualize the oropharynx and is assessed with the patient sitting in front of the scanner, upright, mouth open to maximum and the maximum protrusion tongue without phonation then assesses the extent visible posterior pharyngeal elements (Figure 1).

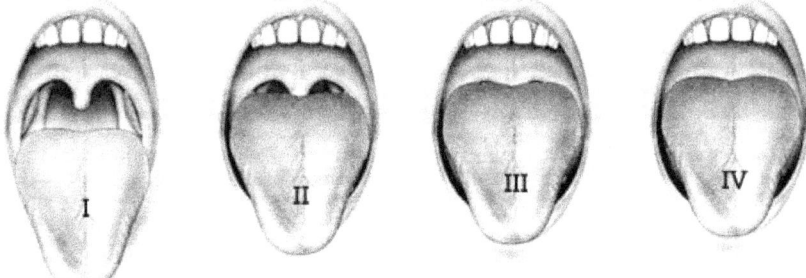

Figure 1 - Classification of the upper airways according to the size of the tongue and oropharyngeal structures (Mallampati et al.)[8,9]

The visualization of these structures is related to the ease or difficulty of laryngoscopy and intubation of the patient (Table 2).

CLASS 1	PILLARS AND VISIBLE UVULA
CLASS 2	SOFT PALATE AND VISIBLE UVULA, UVULA BUT IS HIDDEN BY THE BASE OF THE TONGUE
CLASS 3	SOFT PALATE AND VISIBLE UVULA
CLASS 4	SOFT PALATE NO VISIBLE

Table 2- Clasification of Mallampati.

2 - Classification Patil Aldreti

The space above the larynx determines how easily the laryngeal axis is aligned with the pharyngeal axis when the atlanto-occipital joint is in extension.

If tiromental distance is very short, the laryngeal axis form a more acute angle with the pharyngeal axis, being easy to measure with a ruler or through the width through the fingers, this is known as tiromental distance and / or length horizontally jaw; the classification made by Patil Aldreti evaluates the distance between the thyroid cartilage and the lower edge of the chin, the patient sat with his head in full extension and mouth shut while.[10]

If this distance is greater than 6.5 cm would have no problem. 6 to 6.5 cm, laryngoscopy and intubation difficult, but possible. Less than 6 cm, intubation impossible.

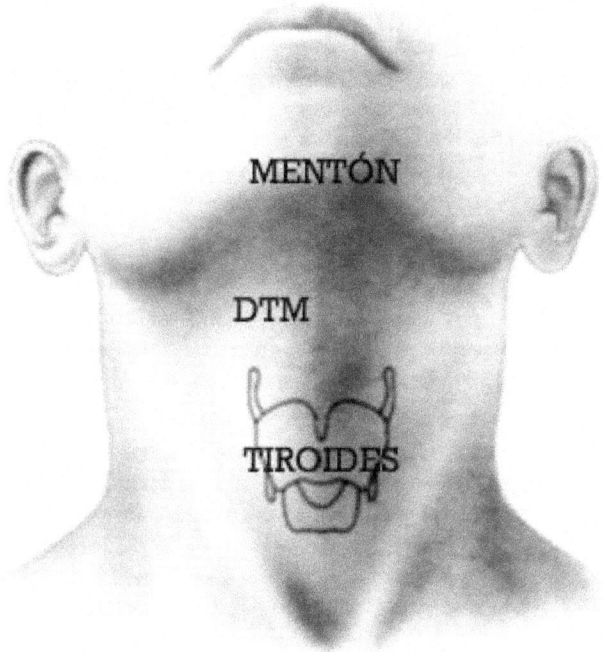

Figure 2 - Distance or thyromental .[10]

2-   Classification Cormack-Lehane.

The visualization by laryngoscopy was defined by Cormack and Lehane and divided into degrees.
Grade I is a complete visualization of the laryngeal aperture; grade

II in the posterior portion of the laryngeal opening is displayed only; grade III is displayed only the epiglottis, and grade IV is displayed only the soft palate (Figure 2).

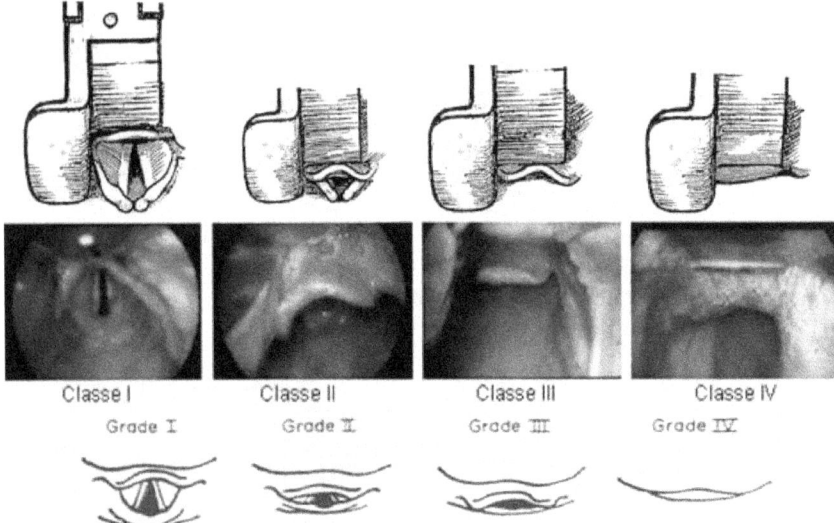

Figure 2 - Grades visualization of the laryngeal opening by laringoscopia (Cormack Lehane).[9]

Medical Jokes: "You know what the students medical Wizards? (A college professor doctor) - not a teacher, what? - Are the therapists or neurosurgeons and intensivists. Why teacher? - Because neurosurgeons transform animal vegetable queen; and intensive vegetable mineral reigns.. "

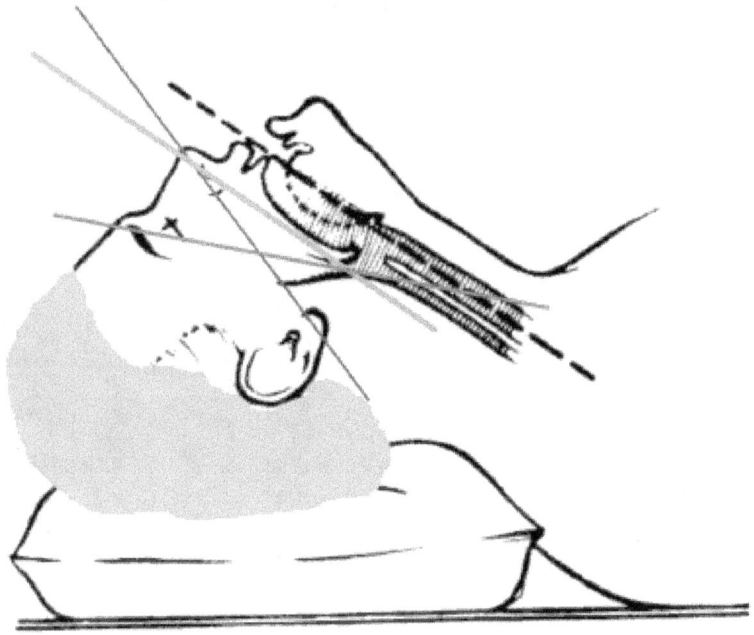

Figure 3 - Alignment of the Axes of the upper airway.

It has been determined that there are 3 parameters that determine the adequate visualization of the larynx: size of the upper incisors, position of the larynx and tongue size (Figure 3).

Direct view of the vocal cords at laryngoscopy can be blocked by a previous larynx; position of the larynx (Cormack and Lehane).[13, 14]

3 - There is another method developed by Belhause and Doré, is the assessment of atlanto-occipital joint, requires a cooperative patient who was not suffered whiplash as the extension or flexion of the neck can cause cervical lesions.

The patient should sit with your head erect, looking ahead and extend the atlanto-occipital joint with a minimum length of the rest of the cervical spine in this position the occlusal surface of the upper teeth is horizontal and parallel to the floor.

Then the patient to extend the joint calls atlanto-occipital as much as possible and the examiner estimates the angle formed by the line through the occlusal surface of the upper teeth and certain previous line, this angle[11, 12] has determined that there should be 35 ° (Figure 4).

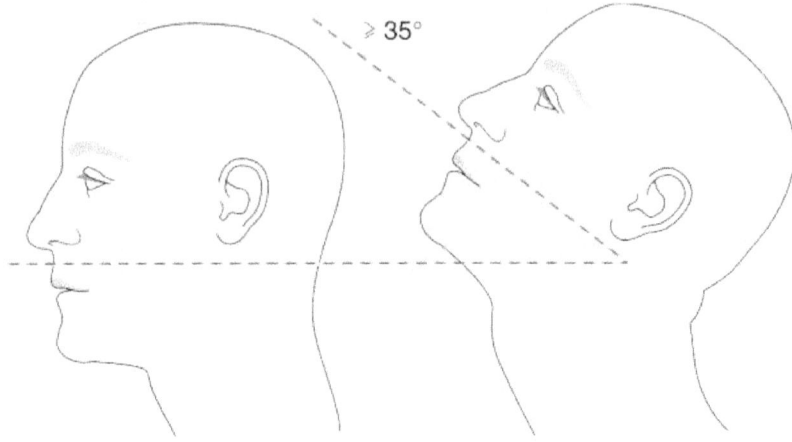

Figure 4 - clinical method for assessing the extent of the atlanto-occipital joint (Belhause and Doré).[11, 12]

Any of the above options can be used to determine if there will be difficult intubation.

CARDIO-RESPIRATORY EXPLORATION

The cardio-respiratory examination includes inspection of the chest to determine the shape, volume, surface condition and movements, followed by auscultation of lung fields to identify acoustic phenomena and the aggregates decreased breath sounds, continue with the exploration of cardiac auscultation area frequency, intensity and rhythm of the heart sounds, lights added in the exploration of the valve system to detect abnormal noise phenomena and the presence of systolic flow murmurs.

Radiologically you can see the heart shadow, as well as pathological images of the aorta and / or deviations or tracheal stenosis.

Either way, whether known or unknown cardiovascular disease, a number of symptoms and signs which have acquired great predictive value for cardiac complications in patients who will be operated such as Goldman multifactorial cardiac index (Table 3).[15, 16, 17]

GOLDMAN		DETSKY	
Item	Ptos	Item	Ptos
Age - 70 years old	5	Age - 70 years old	5
Hearth attack - 6 months	10	Hearth attack - 6 months	10
No sinus rythm or ventricular extrasystoles	7	Hearth attack - 6 months	5
Ventricular extrasystoles -5 per minute	7	Unstable angina - 3 months	10
Jugular venous engorgement or galloping rhythm	11	Pulmonary edema - 1 week	10
Aortic stenosis	3	Pulmonary edema in the past	5
Urgency surgery	4	Sinus rhythm and atrial extrasystoles	5
Chest surgery, abdominal or aorta	3	No sinus rhythm and ventricular extrasystoles	5
Overall organic disease state	3	CCS class III	10
		CCS class IV	20
		Severe aortic stenosis	20
		Urgency surgery	10
		Overall organic disease state	5
Total points possible	53	Total points possible	

Table 3 - Multivariate Índex Goldman.

This index was created in 1977 by Goldman and colleagues from a study in 1,001 patients who would be undergoing non-cardiac surgical procedures, identifying nine major risk factors to which a score was given according to their relative importance in the postoperative mortality cardiac causes (Table 3).

To obtain the total score four risk categories were established, taking into account that the higher the score greater chance of sudden death in the postoperative period; Goldman managed with this data predict the subsequent evolution of 81% of the patients studied.

From the clinical point of view, one way to assess functional capacity obtained through the interrogation is to use the calculated energy requirements for various activities (Figure 5).[18]

1 MET		4 METS
You can do everything alone?		Climb ladders?
Eating, dressing, going to the bathroom alone?		Walk plateau to 4 mph?
Walk inside the home?		Short Run?
Walk 1 or 2 blocks plateau level 2 at 3 mph?		Makes work at home, sweep floors, run furniture?
Makes work at home, clean and wash dishes?		Play golf, bowling, baseball, soccer, or dance?
4 MET		10 METS

Figure 5 - Power requirements for different activities in perioperative cardiovascular evaluation for noncardiac surgery. METS: metabolic equivalents. Taken from Fechner GF. Duke activity status index.

The spine should be explored in its path, especially in the lumbar region and that it is essential to detect deviations and deformities, and skin infections that contraindicate regional anesthesia.[19]

Neurological examination may be brief in healthy people remembering that disease toxemic pregnant patient presents with increased tendon reflexes.

LABORATORY TESTS

Among the most important laboratory tests anesthesiologist should have updated CBC tests.

Other tests such as urinalysis, blood chemistry and coagulation test, if possible, they, with less than 24 hours duration will be requested.

The trend is less evidence request laboratory growing, most of which should be based on patient history.

PULMONARY FUNCTION TESTS

Since the pulmonary function tests are relatively insensitive and expensive, not routinely recommended for smokers and patients with other underlying disease.

In most cases, interrogation, auscultation and chest radiography are sufficient to formulate an anesthetic plan.

8 PRE-OPERATIVE INTERCONSULTATIONS WITH OTHER SPECIALISTS

The pre-operative consultations are classified into two main categories:

1- The cases for which more information or experience is needed to establish a diagnosis or quantify implications for anesthetic management.

2- Patients in whom the diagnosis is known, but further evaluation is needed to optimize treatment for his medical condition prior to surgery for the anesthetic management.

An example of the first type of reference would be to ask a cardiologist who values a 50 year old man with recent onset of chest pain with exertion.

Send patients with diabetes, hypertension or asthma who were not adequately controlled with a clinician is a good example of the second type of query.

Prior to terminate the pre-anesthetic assessment is necessary to make planning more anesthetic method followed in each case the patient explaining the pros and cons of anesthetic technique selected security infusing both surgical and anesthetic staff involved for such end.[20]

It is necessary to emphasize that the success of the pre-anesthetic visit depends fundamentally on the psychological management of anxiety, as the calm and cooperative patient predicts a happy ending.[21, 22]

Medical Jokes:

A patient wakes up after anesthesia, and sees a man on his right and asked, 'Doctor, everything went well in the operation? And the Lord replied: - So, I'm not your doctor, I am St. Peter, and second this is not a hospital, it is heaven.

-Doctor, doctor, I am very nervous, is the first operation that I submit in my life. -Calm down, this is my first anesthetic procedure ...

Doctor in a hospital emergency: Mr. Cosme-Family! -If we are. -We will need an plate for your family. - Radiological doctor? -No, marble.

-Doctor, can have children after 40? -Personally, lady, I think forty children is enough ...

9 CONCLUSION

The pre - anesthetic assessment clinics in hospitals and low complexity is the essential element or tool of anesthetic management of the patient.

The practice environment may have an important role in the type of patient and procedure but should not decrease the quality of care in a given patient.

The doctor will do a good patient triage to know what will benefit and can be operated in hospitals and clinics low complexity , depending on a good pre- operative assessment , always taking into account the health and safety integrity.

Address is not recommended anesthetic procedures in hospitals and clinics with low complexity ASA III patients (three) , nor surgeries very long time and a lot of fluid exchange .

Keep in mind that the need for blood is always latent , and not risk embarking on surgery or suspected have significant bleeding , but we have a logistical support of blood .

Write, write, write and always; all patient data, both in the pre-anesthetic, assessment as well as on leaf anesthesia in the operating room, often taking all registered medico legal problems are avoided and help other colleagues in the team to know conclusively that it was performed a particular patient. For example to make clear an unanticipated difficult intubation, etc..

Always remember that all anesthetic procedure can get complicated, so be prepared with all the tools at hand.

Fernando Martín Correa

10 REFERENCES

1- American Society of Anesthesiologyst. New classification of physical status anesthesiology. Estados Unidos, 1963, 24:111.
2- Pasternak LR. The task force on pre anesthesia evaluation. Practice advisory for pre anesthesia evaluation. Anesthesiology 2002; 96: 485-96.
3- American Society of Anesthesiologyst. Basic standars for pre anesthesia care. Guidelines and statements. 2002. p.s.
4- American Society of Anesthesiologyst. Guidelines for ambulatory anesthesia and surgery. Guidelines and Statements, section II A. 2002. p. 18.
5- Haberkrn Ch M y Lecky J H. Evaluación pre-operatoria y la clínica de la anestesia. En: Clínicas de Anestesiología de Norteamérica. México, Interamericana, Vol. 4, 1996, 554-555.
6- Leonel Canto Sanchez. Anesthesia obstétrica. Manual Moderno, México, 2001; 5: 52.
7- López A. Fundamentos de Anestesiología. La prensa médica Mexicana, 1988, 1-15.
8- Mallampati SR, Gatt SP et al. A clinical sign to predict difficult tracheal intubation. A retrospective study. Can Anaesth Soc J, 1985; 32:429.
9- Sansoon GL, Young SR. Difficult tracheal intubation: a retrospective study. Anesthesia 1987; 42-487.
10- Rocke DA, Murray W. Relative risk analysis of factors associated with difficult intubation in obstetric anesthesia. Anesthesiology 1992; 77: 67-73.
11- ASA Practice Guidelines for Management of the difficult Airway, Anesthesiology 1993; 78: 597-602.
12- Wilson E, Spiegelhater D, Robertson JA, Lesser P. Predicting

difficult intubation. Br J Anesthesiol. 1988; 61: 211-216.

13- Wikinski J. La visita preanestésica. En: Aldrete J. Anestesiología teórico-práctica. Salvat, 1994: 333-357.

14- Baduer N, Nielson W, Munk S et al. Preoperative anxiety: Detection and contributing factors. Can J Anaesth 1990; 37:414.

15- Detsky AS, Abrams HB et al. Predecting cardiac complications in patients undergoing non-cardiac surgery. J Intern Med 1986; 4:211.

16- Goldman L, Multifactorial risk index at ten years. Anesthesiology 1987; 1: 231.

17- Fleisher L. Evaluación Preoperatoria. En: Barash P. Anestesia Clínica. Mc Graw-Hill Interamericana, 1988:523-542.

18- Pastor Luna, Anestesia en el Cardiópata. Mc Graw-Hill Interamericana, 2004: 13.

19- Morgan E, Mikhail M. Anestesiología Clínica. Editorial El Manual Moderno, México, 1995: 741-777.

20- Clínicas de Anestesiología. Valoración Preoperatoria. Mc Graw-Hill Interamericana, 2004, 4: 129-140.

21- James Duke, M.D., Secretos de la Anestesia. Segunda Edición. Mc Graw-Hill Interamericana, México, 2003; III: 85-94.

22- Miguel Angel Paladino y col. Farmacología para Anestesiólogos e Intensivistas. Fundación Anestesiológica de Rosario, Argentina, 2001: 19-84.

23- www.fibroanestesia.com. Web médica acreditada.

24- http://anestesiologos.blogspot.com

ABOUT THE AUTHOR

The author of this work became a doctor at the National University of Cordoba, Argentina. He completed his medical residency in anesthesiology at the National Hospital Itauguá, Anesthesiology graduate of the National University of Asuncion; is currently an anesthesiologist at the Central Hospital of IPS, Itauguá National Hospital and Regional Hospital of Luque, Paraguay.
Also as guardian of anesthesiology residents in these hospitals and resident coordinator of the second year of graduate Anesthesiology dependent IPSC Catholic University of Asuncion.

www.ingramcontent.com/pod-product-compliance
Lightning Source LLC
Chambersburg PA
CBHW070721180526
45167CB00004B/1568